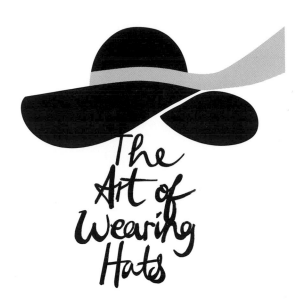

The
Art of
Wearing
Hats

For Rhodri and Caroline

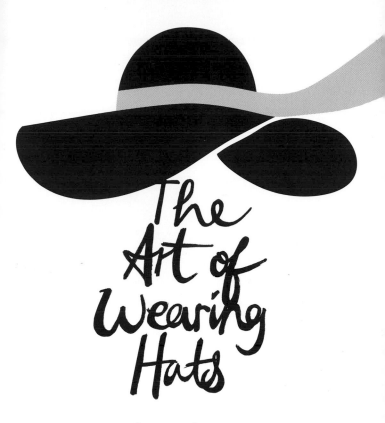

The Art of Wearing Hats

**What to choose
Where to find
How to style**

—

Helena Sheffield

HarperCollins*Publishers*

HarperCollins*Publishers*
1 London Bridge Street
London SE1 9GF

www.harpercollins.co.uk

First published by HarperCollins*Publishers* 2016

1 3 5 7 9 10 8 6 4 2

© Helena Sheffield 2016

Illustrations © Sian Tezel

Helena Sheffield asserts the moral right to be
identified as the author of this work

A catalogue record of this book is
available from the British Library

HB ISBN 978-0-00-816529-1
EB ISBN 978-0-00-816536-9

Printed and bound in China

MIX
Paper from
responsible sources
FSC™ C007454

FSC is a non-profit international organisation established to promote the
responsible management of the world's forests. Products carrying the FSC
label are independently certified to assure consumers that they come from
forests that are managed to meet the social, economic and ecological
needs of present and future generations and other controlled sources.

Find out more about HarperCollins and the environment at
www.harpercollins.co.uk/green

Contents

—

No.4:
Tricks of the **Trade**

Introduction

—

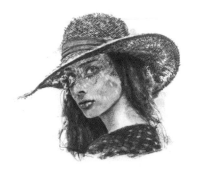

The hat is back. Not with a bang
or a grandiose flourish, but with
a growing murmur as it gathers a
dedicated following. It's cropping up
more and more frequently: from
weddings and walks, to festivals,
holidays and quick nips to the shops,
people are rediscovering the trilby
and the turban, the pillbox and
the pork pie. It's a quietly quirky
fashion revolution.

Do you want to know a secret? The hat never left. While it's been fading from common use over the past few decades, every now and then someone rediscovers it. Look at Kate Middleton, Cara Delevingne, Justin Timberlake and Pharrell Williams: all lauded for their pioneering hattitude, and all inspiring more and more people to don a hat.

This book is an ode to you – to the person who sees the power of a good hat, whether they wear one or not. If you're already a hat enthusiast, delve into these pages for ideas to further refine your unique look. If you're afflicted by The Fear, believing that hats don't suit you, ask yourself why that is – it's possible that you simply haven't found the right one yet.

Catwalking some of the best, most versatile hats around, this book offers advice on how and when to wear them, what with and where to, and lists a variety of shops to buy them from. It suggests which hats suit different face shapes and head sizes, and gives tips and tricks for making the most of each hat. It provides stories from the history of different hats (you might be surprised by some), and will point you in the direction of becoming the hat-wearer you were always born to be.

Wearing a hat doesn't actually take anything more than confidence, but understanding the true magic of hats – and how they can transform the wearer into a mysterious stranger – can't always be learnt alone. Using this book will help you uncover their secrets, master them and work out how to wear hats every day.

How
to Use
This Book

—

The list of contents and index in this book can help you determine exactly what kind of hat you're looking for, with the contents organising them by occasion and the index by season.

Once you've decided on a hat of interest, you can find more information on its origin, anecdotes from its history and a list of specific suggestions and ideas for finding and wearing it under the following headings:

WEAR IT
When to wear the hat – occasions, weather and season.

OWN IT
What face shapes, head sizes or hair styles can really own the hat.

STYLE IT
What to wear it with.

FIND IT
Where's best to buy one.

PERFECT IT
Top tips and tricks for wearing the hat.

STYLE GURU
Which celebrities wear this hat best and why, giving you all the hat-spiration you'll ever need.

This book is a guide to help you along the path of discovering hats, to encourage you to create your own style and to become an inspiration to the rest of us.

While there are considerably more hats designed for women, this book also provides pointers for those fashion-savvy men who really know how to dress. Many of the hats listed here can – and should! – be adopted by both sexes.

Once you properly start wearing hats, it naturally follows that you'll become an icon. (I know, it's a hard life.) There are burdens that come with such responsibility, and the final section of this book covers common issues faced by hat-wearers today, with a few simple solutions. By dipping in and out of these pages you will become a fully fledged hat-wearer, who commands respect and answers to no one.

A Brief
History
of Hats

—

3,300 BC – The earliest known version of a hat is preserved alongside its owner in the ice of a mountain on the border of Austria and Italy, proving that even in the Bronze Age people knew how to dress. Or just keep their heads warm.

3,200 BC – Tomb paintings depict Egyptian men wearing conical straw hats or headdresses.

AD 800 – St Clement, English patron saint of hatmakers, accidentally discovers felt. You could say that this occurrence ranks alongside similar accidental discoveries, such as penicillin and the Slinky.

1571 – An Act of Parliament is passed decreeing that people over the age of six must wear a hat on Sundays. Of course, this only applies to the 'commoners'.

1597 – The above law is revoked for being far too ridiculous.

17th century – The term 'milliner' is first used to describe hatmakers. Milan is already considered a centre of fashion, so the term suggests that only 'Milan-ers' make hats.

18th century – The French Revolution makes hats unpopular in France (perhaps for the first and last time), as they're seen to indicate social status. It's deemed fashionable – and safer – to appear democratic, so hats drop out of use.

19th century – Women's necks are considered too erotic for public display, so bonnets are fashioned with frills and ribbons at the back to cover them up.

1914–1918 – During the First World War fabric is scarce, so plumes of feathers and overly adorned hats are frowned upon for being unpatriotic. Hats become much smaller and simpler.

1920s – Women's necks are apparently still considered erotic, as they're all being shown off by shocking new hairstyles and hats that accentuate their length.

1939–1945 – In complete contrast to the First World War, hats are one of the only items of clothing not affected by severe rationing. In France berets are adopted as a symbol of resistance against Nazi occupation, and explosions of feathers and flowers are admired rather than shunned.

Late 1960s – Fashions begin leaning towards the daring young people, and hats gradually fall from grace, perceived as the preserve of older, more conservative dressers.

2011 – The wedding of the century takes place between Prince William and Kate Middleton, bringing the hat back with resounding success. Royalty and guests wear hats with panache, style and unfailing confidence, finally returning them to the public eye.

2016 – A book so brilliant, useful and witty is published, championing the hat and inspiring a revolution of new hat-wearers, that it will later be heralded as the tome that changed the fashion industry for good. (Clue: you're reading it.)

Hats
to Wear
Every
Day

№1

'I myself have twelve hats, and each one represents a different personality. Why just be yourself?'

—

Margaret Atwood

The
TRILBY

—

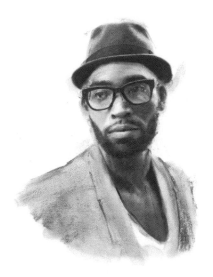

This hat was famously inspired by Trilby O'Ferrall, a character from one of George du Maurier's novels who, in a stage adaptation, wore an interesting new soft hat that was quickly named after her and adopted by the public in the late 19th century. It has always been more popular in America than in Britain, and because of this is often confused for a fedora – a grave mistake indeed!

WEAR IT: ANYWHERE AND EVERYWHERE
This hat suits day and night during autumn and winter. Always smart, it's one both men and women can wear with ease.

OWN IT: BIG HAIR, LONG FACES
As it's a narrow hat, the trilby suits long faces best. It also works well with big hair as the material is soft and flexible.

STYLE IT: CRISP SHIRT AND TROUSERS
The trilby means business, and it therefore works best with smart outfits – think *The Blues Brothers* or Marlene Dietrich.

FIND IT: ALMOST EVERYWHERE
Trilbies can be bought in every hat establishment you can think of – vintage shops, high-street shops, milliners and even fancy-dress shops. You now have no excuse not to get one.

PERFECT IT: DON A WAISTCOAT
Whether male or female, this is not only dapper, but authoritative and oh-so-suave.

STYLE GURU
The one and only Justin Timberlake has displayed a wealth of trilbies over the years. The smooth-talking singer often wears them with a Suit & Tie, and that's Not a Bad Thing.

The
BOWLER

—

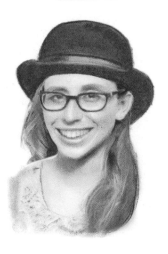

The world's first bowler hat was made for a game-keeper in 1849, and the first thing he did when he saw it was jump on it. No, that wasn't out of disgust, but to check whether it could support his weight and thus be suitable for wearing in all weathers. Although originally meant for withstanding the sharp winds and torrential rain of the British countryside, it was quickly adopted by city workers in Britain and America before falling out of regular use in the 1960s. An easier-to-wear, modern version has recently exploded back onto the scene, making the bowler a distinctly stylish hat once more.

WEAR IT: IN THE DRY OR THE DAMP
Because bowler hats are tight-fitting, the wind can't blow them off your head (a common and harrowing problem that will be addressed in Chapter 4), and their tough felt material isn't bothered by a bit of rain.

OWN IT: SMALL HEADS AND ROUND FACES
Modern incarnations of the hat are fashioned to rest primly atop your head, suiting round faces in particular. They're not big hats, so smaller heads benefit from this.

STYLE IT: BLACK SKINNY JEANS, A STRIPED TOP AND A BOWLER
This look is not only embarrassingly easy to put together, but also gives a classic twist to a popular outfit.

FIND IT: HIGH STREET
Bowler hats are everywhere. You'll find one in most big high-street shops from autumn through to spring.

PERFECT IT: ALL NIGHT LONG
Swap trainers for smart shoes to go from a stylish day-time to a polished evening look.

STYLE GURU
Fearne Cotton, a respected hat champion, often nails the bowler, teamed with a simple, 'thrown-together' look and a dash of lipstick.

The
CLOCHE

—

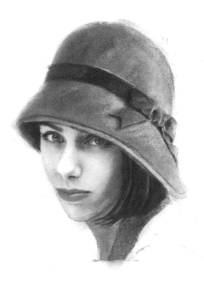

The 1920s is perhaps the only era defined by a hat. The cloche – chic, stylish and simple – was created by French milliner Caroline Reboux. By 1924 the cloche had transfixed the continent, even inspiring novels such as *The Green Hat*, which became known as the book that encapsulated the frenzied hysteria of the decade. Snuggly skimming the nape of the neck, the cloche creates an elegant, elongated line that evokes nostalgia for a time long past.

WEAR IT: DAY OR NIGHT
One of the most versatile of hats, it never fails to deliver a final splash of panache to every outfit.

OWN IT: CROPPED HAIR
On account of its structured shape the cloche is fairly rigid, and it might be difficult to wear one if you have big hair. A cropped haircut is neat and will peek out from beneath like a secret begging to be discovered.

STYLE IT: FULL SKIRTS AND FLOATY DRESSES
Although originally worn with the slim-fitting, scandalous dresses of the 1920s, the cloche is great for balancing the flare of big skirts with its graceful shape.

FIND IT: INDEPENDENT HAT SHOPS
While high-street shops are starting to adopt the cloche, independent hat shops have a real variety of colours and styles to help you find your unique hat.

PERFECT IT: THROW ON A CAPE
It might sound strange, but instead of putting on a coat in the winter try wearing a cape, letting it lend that extra element of dignity that the cloche completes. It's also particularly fun to swoosh around in . . .

STYLE GURU
Check out Angelina Jolie in *The Changeling* for hats that will change your world for the better.

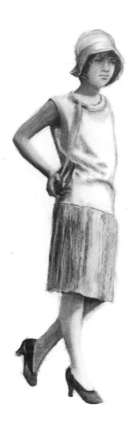

'A well-dressed woman, even though
her purse is painfully empty, can
conquer the world.'

Louise Brooks

GET THE LOOK:
The 1920s

For setting the world on fire with fierce cropped hair and unapologetic lifestyles, women of the 1920s are still idolised today. Draped in beads or furs, their look is not now a practical one, but it can be tweaked to help you achieve that dazzling aura.

THE HAT Any cloche hat will work for this look, but pay attention to detail so you find one that will match one other element of your outfit – be that colour, design or fabric.

THE OUTFIT To achieve the full style, aim for a loose-fitting, drop-waisted dress. This doesn't need to be smart or formal – the beauty of this look is that it's meant to seem like it's simply been thrown on in a slapdash manner.

THE ACCESSORIES A string of pearls and dark red lipstick are all you really need to complete the outfit, but incorporating fur into it will finish it off to perfection. This could be in the form of a coat or cape with fur attached, or a simple fur collar. The latter in particular can be found in various vintage shops.

The
BOATER

—

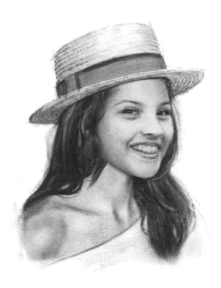

The boater's first foray into fashion was as an informal hat, heralding a new age of wearing hats for leisure. It was worn by men during the summer months in the early 20th century, having previously served as an item of uniform for Victorian schoolchildren (how delightful if that could still be enforced!). It's now most often seen during the famed Henley Royal Regatta every summer, as well as remaining popular in many European countries.

WEAR IT: SUMMERTIME

As an exclusively straw hat, stick to wearing this during the summer. Don't worry about getting caught in the rain, though – the thick straw can easily withstand the wet.

OWN IT: WIDE BRIMS FOR WIDE FACES

Boaters often come with wide brims, meaning they're the right size for wider faces. People with oval or narrow faces should look out for smaller brims to avoid an imbalance.

STYLE IT: SUNGLASSES

The right pair of sunglasses can alter the tone of every outfit. A pair of horn-rimmed or cat-eye glasses will give a vintage feel, while a modern, chunky pair will look more laid-back and casual.

FIND IT: VINTAGE SHOPS

Vintage shops or vintage fairs will have the best choice of boaters. If there are none near you, try looking online.

PERFECT IT: PACK UP YOUR TROUBLES

Which hat should you take on holiday? The boater, without question. Place it upside down in your suitcase, pack it neatly with smaller items (socks and underwear are perfect), and then pack your clothes around it. It will hardly take up any room.

STYLE GURU

Leonardo DiCaprio's turn as Jay Gatsby meant boaters aplenty – and oh, how he wore them . . .

The
MILITARY
CAP

—

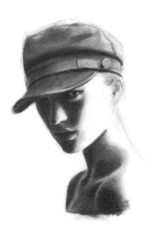

Throughout history the military has had an excellent record of innovative and stylish headgear, including that most swashbuckling of hats, the tricorne. This was originally created by sailors who turned up their brims to funnel rainwater away from their faces. The style was adopted by the French, who proceeded to add brocade and feathers to glam it up, and tricornes were worn by naval officers throughout the 18th century. The style of 'military cap' in current fashion is a soft-peaked cap (unfortunately nothing like the tricorne), and it's surprisingly simple to wear.

WEAR IT: DURING THE DAY
This hat is neat and practical, so is perfect to wear while out and about during the day.

OWN IT: IF YOU'RE A LITTLE HAT SHY
The military cap isn't garish and doesn't get in the way. If you're finding hats difficult or cumbersome, then try this one – you'll almost forget it's there.

STYLE IT: WITH A JACKET
The jacket here means everything. A military jacket maintains the theme and implies that you're just this close to joining the Army; a leather jacket makes it much more casual (and is undeniably cool); and a blazer smartens it up but creates a softer image than the military jacket.

FIND IT: ONLINE
These are harder to find than most, but there are many excellent examples that can be found online.

PERFECT IT: PUT YOUR HAIR UP
The soft material means it's one of the few hats that can actually be worn with your hair tied up underneath it (try a bun for minimal bulkiness).

STYLE GURU
Rihanna has been known to rock a military hat. Regardless of her hairstyle, she makes them look fierce and unforgettable.

The
PORK
PIE

—

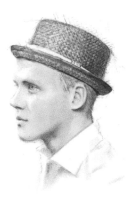

Although generally known as a hat for men, the pork pie hat was originally introduced as women's fashion in Britain and America around 1830. It wasn't until Buster Keaton adopted it as his signature hat in the 1920s that it became popular with men. There's debate about the origins of the name 'pork pie'. (Yes, we debate these things. Yes, you too will soon want to debate about hats.) Some say it's because the short brim and crease around the crown make it look like a pork pie, others that the hats were made using pie tins as moulds. Either way, the pork pie is a tasty addition to your hat collection.

WEAR IT: ALL YEAR
Available in felt and straw, you can prepare yourself for all seasons. It's more unique than the bowler, so can also be worn at special occasions.

OWN IT: NARROW/OVAL FACES
The pork pie is made of very stiff material and is meant to sit towards the back of your head. While this can make it difficult to wear for some, it perfectly complements narrower or oval face shapes and simple hairstyles.

STYLE IT: EMBRACE THE KNITWEAR
A thick, brightly patterned wool jumper will contrast splendidly with this quiet hat.

FIND IT: VINTAGE SHOPS
Pork pies are not always easy to find, but you should have success in vintage shops or proper hat shops.

PERFECT IT: LESS IS MORE
This is an understated hat, and too many accessories can distract from it. Wear it with a simple outfit as the only embellishment to really make it stand out.

STYLE GURU
Bryan Cranston has brought the pork pie back with criminal success by playing Walter White in the beloved *Breaking Bad* series.

WIDE-BRIMMED HATS

—

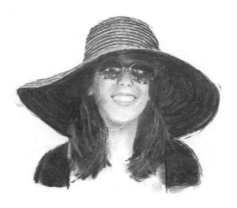

You'll never know when you're ready to wear a wide-brim, so the best thing to do is to plunge yourself into it head first (quite literally), with no regrets. You might worry that it's entirely out of place, but no one else will think so – they're likely to be suffering from hat lust and wishing they had your confidence. A wide-brimmed hat will get you noticed, but it also gets in the way, blows off in the wind and is a nightmare to pack or travel in. It's essentially a high-risk, high-reward hat.

You might be wondering why you should bother. They're so big, so cumbersome. There are two words to clarify this: Audrey Hepburn. If you've seen *that* hat in *Breakfast at Tiffany's*, you'll understand the unparalleled sophistication it lends her. Wide-brimmed hats change the way you hold yourself, the way you walk, even the way you feel. You could probably save the world in that hat.

WEAR IT: WHEN THERE'S NO WIND
Wind is a serious hazard to a wide-brim. Otherwise you can wear it all year round, and especially to turn heads at smart or formal occasions.

OWN IT: WITH CONFIDENCE
The key to wearing a wide-brim successfully is nothing to do with head size or face shape: the only trick is your confidence.

STYLE IT: GO VINTAGE
Wear them with mid-length skirts or dresses for a touch of 1940s glamour, or a brightly patterned jump-suit and big sunglasses to give your look a 1970s spin.

FIND IT: HIGH STREET
High-street shops have a huge number of wide-brimmed hats available all year, so these are the best places for your first one. To branch out, try independent hat shops and vintage fairs.

PERFECT IT: BEWARE OF BLINDNESS
If you're choosing a straw wide-brim, try to find one that isn't too floppy; no one wants impeded vision!

STYLE GURU
Audrey Hepburn in *Breakfast at Tiffany's* (she should also be your guru in general life). She's simply the queen of the wide-brimmed hat.

Hats
to Wear
in the
Wild

Nº2

'Hats are a great antidote to what's going on. It's really their purpose to put a happy face on a sad world ... That's the thing about hats. They're extravagant and full of humour and allow for a sense of costume, but in a lighthearted way.'

—

Stephen Jones

The
BERET

—

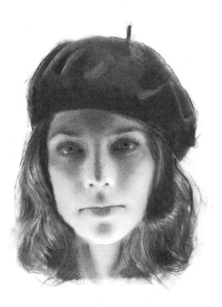

An issue facing prospective hat-wearers today is the
sheer variety available. How to choose between a flat
cap and a trilby, a cloche and a riding cap? The answer
is simple: start with the basics. The beret is a decep-
tive and therefore most underrated hat. It has become
a caricature atop the head of a moustachioed French-
man wearing a string of onions, but its benefits often
go ignored.

WEAR IT: ON A BLUSTERY DAY
The beret is naturally adept at keeping out the cold and not getting blown off your head. It's an ideal autumnal hat, but the range of colours and styles make it suitable most of the year round.

OWN IT: ANYONE AND EVERYONE
The magic of a beret is that it can be worn in any style at any time, so suiting all hair styles and face shapes.

STYLE IT: FOR EVERY SEASON
If it's spring and you want a hat that won't encumber you, pack a cream beret in your bag to whip out at any moment. If it's autumn, pop a plum-coloured beret on your head to prevent cold ears – the beret has them covered.

FIND IT: HIGH STREET
It's almost impossible *not* to find a beret; they're stocked in most high-street shops and are extremely affordable.

PERFECT IT: CREATE A COLOURFUL COLLECTION
Building up a wide range of colours in your beret collection will see you through most of the year and is the perfect way to boost your hat-wearing confidence.

STYLE GURU
Iconic French actress Brigitte Bardot wore a black beret with thick black eyeliner to contrast with her flowing blonde hair. She wore one unapologetically and with serious style.

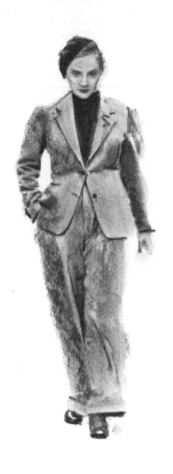

'I dress for the image. Not for myself, not for the public, not for fashion, not for men.'

Marlene Dietrich

GET THE LOOK: The 1930s

Women's fashion in the 1930s was perhaps more scandalous than that of the 1920s: androgyny was everything. Notable Hollywood stars turned up to parties in top hats, came coiffed in Cossacks and wowed with wide-brims. The woman who epitomised this decade was Marlene Dietrich, and one of her well-known looks was a beret and tweed suit – still relevant and achievable today.

THE HAT Marlene chose a black beret, but while you can select any colour to best complement your outfit, make sure to wear it like she did: firmly slanted across one side of your head.

THE OUTFIT As a leading light of the 1930s, Marlene wore high-waisted, wide-legged trousers with most of her outfits. These are readily available today, so match them with a cream shirt or blouse, buttoned to the top, and a jacket. Tweed might not be so easy to find, so try a structured jacket to contrast with the loosely fitting trousers.

THE ACCESSORIES The pin-curled hair of the 1930s was a trademark look but is not easy to do in a hurry. Sweeping your hair into a low ponytail or bun will achieve the same slick, polished look.

The
BEANIE

—

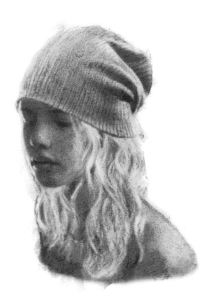

If you had to guess which modern hat was linked to medieval religious tradition, chances are you wouldn't choose the beanie! But way back in 16th-century Wales it was called a Monmouth hat, and a law was passed decreeing that people over six must wear the hat on Sundays and public holidays. Now, don't you think we'd all be better off if there were more laws enforcing weekly hat-wearing?

WEAR IT: WHEN THERE'S A NIP IN THE AIR
It's tight-fitting and snug, so perfect for enduring cold weather. Best worn during the day, the beanie is also perfect for chilly nights out during the winter.

OWN IT: ONE FOR ALL
This is the ultimate androgynous hat that suits all face shapes, head sizes and hair lengths.

STYLE IT: DRAW ATTENTION TO IT
Throwing on a neon-yellow beanie with whatever outfit you're wearing will make more of an impact than any amount of planning. It's the easiest, most accessible and underplayed hat you could hope for.

FIND IT: HIGH STREET
The beanie is readily available on the high street throughout the year.

PERFECT IT: DON'T OVERTHINK IT
This hat hardly needs to be styled. The more flippantly it's worn, the better.

STYLE GURU
Cara Delevingne cannot go unmentioned. She has brought the beanie back into the public eye with power, playfulness and pride.

The
RIDING
HAT

—

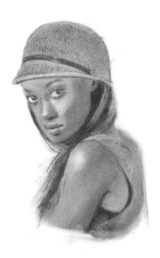

In the Victorian and Edwardian eras, men and women's riding hats were usually top hats – men's tall and made of silk, women's adorned with smart veils and the occasional feather. Nowadays, top hats as riding hats are a victim of health and safety. (It's a travesty. Honestly, wouldn't you risk a fatal head injury so you can gambol about on a horse, a fine top hat affixed to your head?) However, modern riding hats have been widely imitated in the fashion world, which somewhat makes up for this heinous crime.

WEAR IT: IN THE WIND, DAY AND NIGHT
Simple and slim-fitting, this hat is excellent for wearing in blustery weather as the wind can't easily whip it off your head.

OWN IT: NARROW/OVAL FACES
Like the cloche, the riding hat can be quite structured. It best suits smaller face shapes, and can be harder to wear if you've got big hair.

STYLE IT: A BLOUSE AND MID-LENGTH PENCIL SKIRT
Try this for a neat, sophisticated look, and throw on a necktie to add a pinch of 1940s glamour. High-waisted jeans and a buttoned shirt tied at your midriff will convey a more laid-back effect.

FIND IT: INDEPENDENT HAT SHOPS
The finest riding hats can be found in independent or small chain shops – try boutiques, vintage shops and proper hat shops for more quirky variations.

PERFECT IT: BOLD AND BRIGHT
The best way to make the most of this hat is to choose a bold colour. Bright red or mustard yellow will stand out, and are also two colours that should match the blues, greys and blacks in most outfits.

STYLE GURU
Taylor Swift has been upping her hat game and does particularly well with the riding hat. It suits her pixie-like features and country-girl aura.

The
DEERSTALKER

—

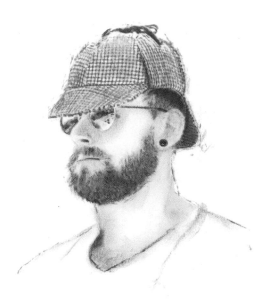

The number of hats with literary connections is large, and the deerstalker is undoubtedly one of these. Famously worn by Sherlock Holmes, it's a curiously designed hat. What on earth possessed someone to fashion those flaps at the back and sides? In fact, the truth is simply that the flaps were meant to warm the ears and neck while men were out shooting, but could be tied up if they got in the way.

WEAR IT: TO BATTLE THE ELEMENTS
Designed to protect heads everywhere from the outside world, the deerstalker does the job of keeping you warm, but also makes a statement.

OWN IT: SMALL FACES
The deerstalker is a compact hat (making it excellent for travel purposes), and it won't overshadow smaller faces.

STYLE IT: LAYER UP
Wearing it with a wax coat would keep you warm and toasty all over, but alternatively a leather jacket might actually make it look very cool indeed.

FIND IT: INDEPENDENT HAT SHOPS
Deerstalkers don't feature on the high street as often as other hats so seek them out in specialist hat shops, which are more likely to stock them. If you're struggling, try street markets – they often have a more quirky selection of hats.

PERFECT IT: KNICKERBOCKERS?
During the height of its popularity in the 1870s, men wore the deerstalker with knickerbockers. Perhaps you're the person to revive this fashion ...

STYLE GURU
Benedict Cumberbatch couldn't avoid donning the deerstalker for his role as Sherlock Holmes, and it has since become synonymous with him.

The
FLAT
CAP

—

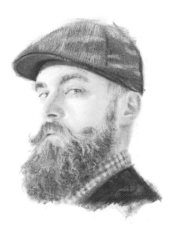

You don't need to be a farmer or be stitched up in tweed to wear a flat cap. Its beauty lies in its ability to evoke a country tone wherever you are, without needing to trudge around town in muddy wellies with a flock of sheep following you. Despite its country connotations, the flat cap first gained popularity in cities and was the hat of choice for the 'working man', before being adopted by the Bright Young Things of the 1920s. What with tweed and Barbour jackets now making a comeback, the flat cap is set to burst into mainstream fashion once again.

WEAR IT: WHEN IT'S SUNNY
The peak of the flat cap actually provides a bit of shade for your eyes if the sun's out. It's definitely more of an autumn and winter hat, and good to bear in mind for those few bright, sunny days in December.

OWN IT: SHORT HAIR OR LONG FACES
Long, oval faces benefit from this style, as it doesn't elongate the face but rather frames it. People with short hair shouldn't hesitate to don a flat cap, as it's one of the few hats that really shows off their hairstyle. Women with bobbed hair might struggle, however – flat caps sit just above the ears, which can do terrible things to this haircut.

STYLE IT: WHITE BUTTONED SHIRT, TROUSERS AND KNEE-HIGH BOOTS
This will give a clean country look – go for green or purple trousers as a twist, or try a simple denim dress, patterned tights and brogues to make it more casual.

FIND IT: ONLINE
It's easiest to find these online, but you could also try vintage shops, which do tend to stock a few.

PERFECT IT: SMARTEN IT UP
Wear it with a waistcoat, because when is a waistcoat a bad idea?

STYLE GURU
None other than Brad Pitt frequently wears a flat cap. Clearly the man has excellent taste and should be an inspiration to us all.

The
FEDORA

—

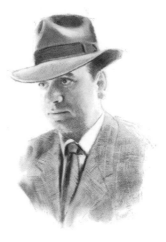

The fedora was inspired by Princess Fédora Romanoff, lead character in a play by Victorien Sardou. When the legendary actress Sarah Bernhardt performed the role wearing this soft-brimmed hat, her fans immediately adopted it. Sound familiar? (See page 18 if not.) It's interesting that the two hats most commonly confused for one another are the two with such similar beginnings. The main difference between the fedora and trilby is the size of the brim: trilbies traditionally have stiff, short brims, while fedoras are much wider. The fedora was popular among women's rights activists in the early 20th century, so it's perhaps ironic that it's known more as a man's hat.

WEAR IT: IN THE RAIN
The large brim and durable felt material means it's a great substitute for an umbrella (well, almost).

OWN IT: BIG HAIR, ROUND FACES
Because of the wide brim, fedoras are particularly good for round or square face shapes. They often come in larger sizes than dainty cloches and riding hats, so big-haired readers, this is the one for you!

STYLE IT: BAGGY SHIRT, SKINNY JEANS, SUNGLASSES
Oh, you think I look effortlessly cool? Why, I just tumbled out of bed and threw this on. It's no big deal ...

FIND IT: HIGH STREET
Fedoras have always had major appeal and most high-street shops stock them in a variety of colours – black, brown and tan are the most common.

PERFECT IT: SUMMERTIME STYLE
Straw fedoras are becoming more common for the summer. If you're pursuing a cowboy look, try it with a checked shirt and shorts (but maybe leave out the leather boots during the heat of summer).

STYLE GURU
Johnny Depp has worn fedoras for years, channelling the vibe of Humphrey Bogart and other classic Hollywood actors, while adding his own unique twist.

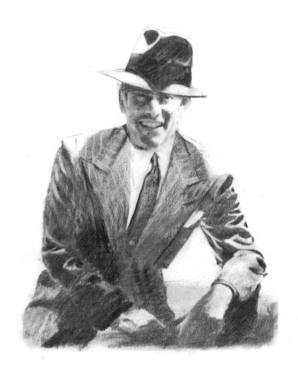

'I believe in dressing for the occasion. There's a time for sweater, sneakers and Levis, and a time for the full-dress jazz.'

Ginger Rogers

GET THE LOOK:
The 1940s

Men's fashion in the 1940s comes across as seriously suave. You could be a New York gangster, a silver-screen star or a survivor of wartime Britain and still know how to strut your stuff in these simple outfits.

THE HAT A simple fedora, no twists or embellishments. These men didn't need anything else to demonstrate that they knew what style was, and neither do you.

THE OUTFIT Nothing says Forties like a fine suit and trench coat, but if that's not your style (you have to play you, after all), how about a shirt and knitted tank top? The former suggests brooding Hollywood actor, the latter vintage geek chic, so really there's nothing to lose.

THE ACCESSORIES If you have a breast pocket, tuck a handkerchief into it to finish off the look. You could also try adding braces, or swapping a tie for a bow tie.

The
COSSACK

—

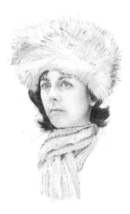

The Cossacks are a Slavic people with perhaps the best hat-based philosophy that has ever been dreamt up. Their hats – papakhas – are connected to their honour, and they have various sayings dedicated to them. The best, and one that ought to be taken to heart even today, states: 'If you have no one to consult, consult your hat.' The papakha has come to be known as the Cossack hat, and is an unashamedly regal addition to your hat collection. If you do happen to be found talking to your hat, you can claim that you're merely honouring a great tradition.

WEAR IT: IN THE MIDST OF WINTER
Made of fur – real or faux – Cossacks are an ideal option for winter months. They're easy to tuck away

in a bag, as they don't take up much room, and are the most fabulous way of keeping your head warm.

OWN IT: ROUND OR FLAT
Cossacks can be rounded or flat-topped. Try a rounded top if you have a smaller, more petite face to allow it to fit more snugly.

STYLE IT: GO RUSSIAN
To channel the Cossacks, wear the hat with a military coat or jacket. If you're after a more dramatic look, try a mid-length 1950s-style skirt or dress to achieve a sweeping, romantic movement, à *la* Anna Karenina.

FIND IT: HIGH STREET
High-street shops tend to offer a variety of colours, but if you're looking for something unique try browsing vintage shops. It's worth bearing in mind that vintage Cossacks are likely to be made from real fur.

PERFECT IT: TO CLASH WITH YOUR HAIR
The Cossack looks best standing out against your hair, so if you're dark-haired choose a white or pale grey hat, and if you're blonde try a black or maroon one. Redheads have the best of both worlds, as white, black and grey will all pop against the hair colour.

STYLE GURU
If you want a film with mesmerising hats, watch *Anna Karenina*. In a film of many memorable hats, Keira Knightley's magnificent Cossack is utterly unforgettable.

The
TRAPPER

—

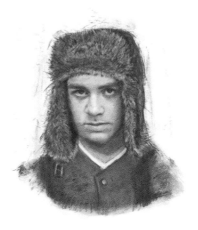

The trapper is a variant of the papakha, but originally used sheep's wool rather than fur to fleece the inside of the hat. Its trademark flaps cover the ears in an arguably more effective way than the deerstalker's, as they too are lined with fur or wool and can be tied under the chin to secure them in place. In 1940 it was adopted by the Soviet Army and sported by its marshals and generals, before becoming more widely worn. Nowadays it makes regular appearances both on catwalks and the high street.

WEAR IT: IN FREEZING WEATHER
This is a more practical hat than the Cossack, particularly for extremely cold environments. The

outside of the hat is often made from tough, sometimes waterproof material, meaning it's one hat that won't be affected by the rain!

OWN IT: IT'S ALL ABOUT FUR
While its variety of shapes and sizes makes this a largely accessible hat, try one with shorter fur if you have a small face, as then it won't shroud you completely.

STYLE IT: LAYER UP
Wearing it with thick leather boots, a fur-lined khaki coat and a chunky jumper will not only make it look like an offhanded afterthought, but will keep you devilishly toasty.

FIND IT: HIGH STREET
An easy hat to find today, it's more likely to be found in high-street shops or online, rather than in vintage shops or milliners.

PERFECT IT: SMARTEN UP
If there's only a nip in the autumn air but you're already eager to get the trapper hat out, wear it with a trench coat to balance out a smart look with a Russian twist.

STYLE GURU
Pharrell Williams, after his recent explosion into the ranks of hat-wearers, has donned a particularly vivid trapper that looks like, well, an explosion ... in the best of ways.

Hats
to Wear
to the
Palace

№3

'I don't use a hat as a prop,
I use it as a part of me.'

—

Isabella Blow

HATINATORS

—

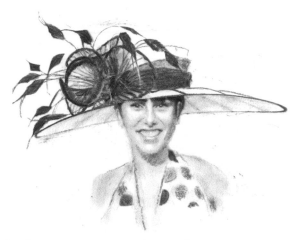

The hatinator section of any department store is nothing short of heaven to hat-wearers. Indeed, seen from a distance, it *could* be taken for heaven, with its vibrant rainbow of colours, plumes of the finest feathers, lace, flowers, veils, ribbons ... It's enough to make one wild with delight.

Hatinators are where milliners truly unleash their creativity, but the opportunities to wear them are few and should be savoured. Buying your first hatinator can seem overwhelming: you want it to dazzle, to provoke intense sensations of hat-lust and feel like an extension of your own being. But how can one piece accomplish so much? The perfect hatinator might not solve all your problems (although it comes close), but it is guaranteed to make you feel like royalty.

WEAR IT: TO WEDDINGS AND FORMAL OCCASIONS
It's tricky to factor the hatinator into everyday life, so save it for special occasions.

OWN IT: TEST YOUR HATINATOR
There are so many sizes available that you will certainly be able to find a hat for your face shape. Those with broad faces could try hats that sit properly on their head rather than perching on a hairband, as they will sit more snugly.

STYLE IT: START WITH THE HAT
Hatinator colours tend to be mostly available in pastels, navy blues and blacks, so choose one before your outfit and coordinate the rest accordingly!

FIND IT: DEPARTMENT STORES
Hatinators are not cheap, but they are widely available in department stores. If you're looking for something absolutely unique, try a milliner or an independent hat shop.

PERFECT IT: BALANCE IT OUT
The bigger and more explosive the hatinator, the simpler your dress should be. Flowers protruding from both hat and dress might induce hay fever and/or overbalance you.

STYLE GURU
Kate Middleton is revered internationally for her dedication to hat-wearing, and her collection of hatinators is nothing short of stunning.

The
TOP HAT

—

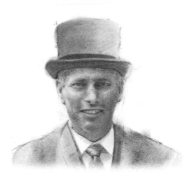

Riots. Terror in the streets. Arresting a man for deliberately scaring timid people. Not the average reaction to a new hat, but in fact a true story about the top hat's first outing. Date? 1797. When milliner James Hetherington sauntered down the street in London in a towering new top hat, crowds gathered to watch, agog and afraid at the horror before them. A police-man arrested him for causing public disorder, but this hat hero had already inspired a generation of outstanding hat-wearers. The top hat is the ultimate piece in high fashion but, alas, it's difficult to find an excuse to wear one of these fine specimens.

WEAR IT: WEDDINGS AND FORMAL OCCASIONS
You know the reality here: top hats are nigh on impossible to wear to work, school, on boats and in the theatre . . . If only they were more practical.

OWN IT: MATCH THE HEIGHT WITH YOUR FACE SHAPE

Long, slim faces are able to pull off the tall, slender style of hat, but if your face is round or square, look out for a shorter height that will complement your face shape.

STYLE IT: TOP HAT AND TAILS

Accompanying a suit and waistcoat, one can rarely wear anything better. It has, however, sometimes been worn along with T-shirts, waistcoats, skinny jeans and a heck of a lot of black eyeliner.

FIND IT: MILLINERS AND HAT SHOPS

Top hats can only really be found in proper hat shops or tailors. They're not cheap, as they're made of a special silk, but if there's one hat to splash the cash on, it's this one.

PERFECT IT: DEFY THE RULES

Every now and again a woman appears on the red carpet in a top hat and tails ... and looks utterly fearsome. It's used as a simple and empowering statement to defy gender stereotypes, and it's all the more stylish for it.

STYLE GURU

Fred Astaire tap-danced in a top hat on many occasions, even starring in a film named *Top Hat*. He is the natural top-hat icon.

The
PILLBOX
HAT

—

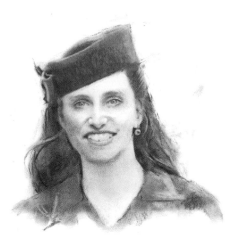

Take a moment to think about Jackie Kennedy. Not only a fashion icon, but a supremely astute and admired woman, she did once make a devastating confession: she didn't like hats. The answer to this problem was presented to her by fashion designer Halston, in the shape of a pillbox hat. With no brim, it was hardly a hat at all – more a piece of headwear that was nonetheless beautiful. Pillboxes enjoyed a relatively short period of popularity from the 1930s to the 1960s, but their simple, elegant designs are gradually making a comeback.

WEAR IT: ANY FORMAL OCCASION

The pillbox is perfect for daytime and evening occasions, and is more suited to winter months than the hatinator, as it's much more durable.

OWN IT: BIG HAIR

If you have big hair with lots of volume, try a larger size and place it firmly on top of your head. If your hair is finer, or you have a narrow or oval face shape, look for a smaller hat and wear it at an angle.

STYLE IT: CHOOSE YOUR ERA

Wear a plain-coloured pillbox with a brightly patterned wrap dress for 1940s chic, or with a simple shift dress and bold liquid eyeliner for Sixties swing. To ooze style, try a pillbox with a small veil attached, and wear bright red lipstick. This will transform an outfit into an artwork and transport you straight back to the 1930s.

FIND IT: INDEPENDENT HAT SHOPS

Some department stores might include pillboxes in their Occasionwear sections, but you'll get more variety in proper hat shops.

PERFECT IT: PIN IT

Pillbox hats used to be fastened with a hatpin. While hatpins are rarely used now, they can be found in antique markets and vintage fairs if you fancy doing things properly.

STYLE GURU

Jackie Kennedy was truly the pillbox pioneer; look to her as an example of excellently effortless hat-wearing.

HATS
WITH
FEATHERS

—

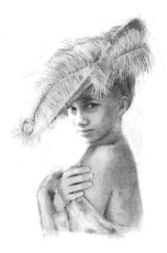

There's little in life so unquestionably refined as a feathered hat. Hats with big, looping bows are all very well, but feathers can be grandiose or subtle, blossoming out of the hat or peeking out, catching the eye of only the most careful observer. There's something about seeing a person in a feathered hat that quite lifts the spirits and sets the heart aflutter.

WEAR IT: IN GOOD WEATHER
Wind or rain can be detrimental to a feathered hat because the feathers, particularly vintage ones, get

damaged very easily. Avoid bad weather if at all possible.

OWN IT: FIND YOUR FAVOURITE
Feathered hats come in any style or shape, so you can easily find the hat that's best for you.

STYLE IT: WITH CONFIDENCE
This kind of hat can get you noticed and help alter the way you feel about yourself. Wearing it to an interview, audition, date or even exam might make all the difference.

FIND IT: VINTAGE SHOPS
While feathered hats are available in most places, you'll find the most unique ones in vintage shops, although these might need to be looked after with extra care.

PERFECT IT: DIY
You can add your own feathers to a hat using a dab of fabric glue in the right place; it's even better if your hat has a bow around the brim, as you can tuck a feather down the side. *Voilà* – your own truly unique hat.

STYLE GURU
If you want a celebrity who has really embraced feathered headpieces, look no further than Lady Gaga. Although her look is not exactly easily achievable, it should certainly be appreciated and admired.

HATS WITH A VEIL

—

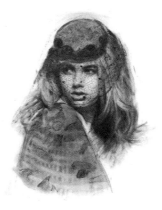

Veils should not be reserved for brides, although if you do wear a veiled hat to a wedding, do be prepared to face a certain level of wrath – it might not end well for you! Weddings aside, wearing hats with veils tends to be reserved for formal occasions, and can be a particularly good option at parties or balls. Veils are mysterious, evoking a Hollywood glamour that will unfailingly make fellow party-goers star-struck, allowing you to swan around in a cloud of compliments.

WEAR IT: EVENING PARTIES OR BALLS
If the event you're wearing a veil to includes food, beware! A veil that covers your full face doesn't make

for easy eating, and starving yourself for the sake of a hat is going a tad far. Make sure you're able to fold or tuck the veil away when it comes to crunch time ...

OWN IT: LOOK OUT FOR A WIDE-BRIM
Veiled hats are usually pillboxes or fascinators, but wider-brimmed hats with veils are making a comeback. These are especially good for round faces.

STYLE IT: DRESS UP
A 1920s flapper dress covered in sequins won't fail to liven up the party, but if you'd like less flair try a sleek black cocktail dress and wait at the bar, Martini in hand, for people to moon over you. They will.

FIND IT: DEPARTMENT STORES
There's usually a good selection of smaller veiled hats in department stores that are more affordable than hatinators. Lots of vintage shops stock them as well, but these will require more upkeep.

PERFECT IT: LOOK AFTER IT
Veiled hats tend to come with other adornments, such as flowers, beads or feathers, making it a tricky hat to pack if you're going away. Have you considered a hat box? If this is too excessive, to protect it wrap it carefully in tissue paper before packing.

STYLE GURU
Princess Diana once wore a veiled riding hat, and it was pure perfection.

The
TURBAN

—

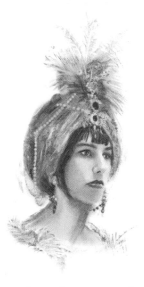

The turban was adopted in Britain for fashion rather than religious purposes in the 17th century. Its English name is derived from variations on the word for tulip, referring to the turban's folds and the way these form layers over each other like tulip petals.

Turbans with swooping feathers and laced with jewels and brocade were fashionable among the more artistic sets in the 1920s, but a simpler style became popular during the 1960s. Its thinner fabric retains the folded character of the classic turban, offering a sleeker but no less noticeable look.

WEAR IT: FOR SPECIAL OCCASIONS
Depending on the style of your turban, it can be worn day or night, but it can be tricky to wear without the right outfit. Try buying one with an outfit in mind to start off with, and build up your confidence from there.

OWN IT: EVERYONE
Turbans mould to your head, so they will suit any face shape. However, if you have a square face and want more height, find one with thicker material that can sit higher up your head.

STYLE IT: WITH SOMETHING SIMPLE
A simple, slim-fitting dress or a mid-length skirt with a blouse is all you need to subtly accentuate it.

FIND IT: VINTAGE SHOPS
Turbans can be hard to come by, and are mainly available in vintage shops. If you're looking for a more show-stopping example, it might be better to try big vintage fairs where there's greater variety.

PERFECT IT: MAKE A STATEMENT
Turbans can be found in all colours imaginable, but to really make an emphatic statement choose one in a bright colour. Bright greens or purples will give a particularly ethnic vibe.

STYLE GURU
Hollywood star Elizabeth Taylor knew how to wear turbans and seriously embraced them, becoming the leader of their resurgence in the Sixties.

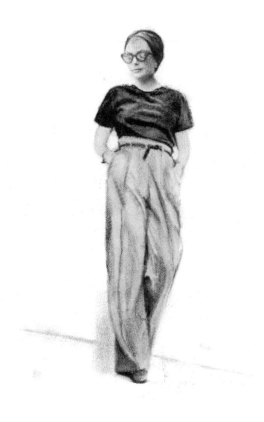

'If anybody starts using me as scenery,
I'll return to New York.'

Grace Kelly

GET THE LOOK:
The 1950s

Grace Kelly was revered throughout the 1950s and beyond. Her most iconic outfit was her wedding dress, which many have since compared to Kate Middleton's in its long-sleeved lace detail and veil. Grace was not averse to donning a turban, however, and if there's anyone who can teach you how to carry it off, it's her.

THE HAT The turbans that best evoke the Grace Kelly aura are the simple 'wrap effect' ones with no embellishments. Try neutral colours such as nude, pale grey or white, which she often adopted to match her clothes.

THE OUTFIT One of Grace's looks is easy to achieve now, and oozes suave sophistication. Match a white turban to a white shirt with blue pinstripes, buttoned to the top, and add navy blue wide-leg trousers.

THE ACCESSORIES To really evoke the 1950s, you need to wear a pair of cat-eye sunglasses. With big, bold frames, these make a statement without you needing to say a word.

Tricks
of the
Trade

Nº4

'How a hat makes you feel is
what a hat is all about.'
—

Philip Treacy

Your
First
Hat

—

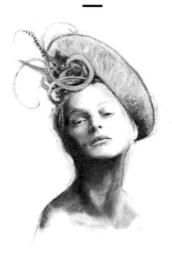

There are so many hats out there in the big, wide world that it's hard to know where to start. In case you're feeling utterly bamboozled at the prospect of beginning your search on your own, here are a few pointers to help you in your choice.

START SMALL, AND WORK WITH AN OUTFIT

Stick to a style you're comfortable with: an outfit you wear often and feel good in will make finding a hat to match it practically effortless, and you can always branch out into other styles later. Choosing a small hat might make your life easier, as you'll almost forget it's there.

WORK UP TO THE WIDE-BRIM

Embracing the wide-brim is a vital part of the journey to becoming a true hat-wearer, but you don't have to dive straight in with any old thing. Keep an eye out for a hat that perfectly suits your style first.

DON'T AGONISE

It might feel like the most important decision you'll ever make, but don't overthink it. If you discover an acid-green hat with plumes of peacock feathers and feel that it speaks to you, then follow your heart and adorn your head with this majestic headpiece.

SUGGESTED STARTING-POINTS

- BERET It won't encumber you with its size, it comes in a variety of colours to match every outfit and it doesn't feel conspicuous.

- BOWLER An easy look to pull off, and a hat that should be a staple of every hat-wearer's wardrobe.

- RIDING HAT Distinguished, quirky and simple enough to work with any outfit.

Building
Your
Confidence

—

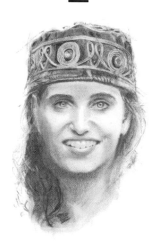

Confidence is what makes you look and feel triumphant inside and out. When embarking upon the noble path of hat-wearing you might come across hats that you don't think you're ready for, but there's one way to conquer your doubts.

The equation for solving any confidence issues you have around hats is simple: (number of hats + time) × 'Who cares what they think' = confidence.

The more hats you have, the more often you're likely to wear them, which will add up to a good few hours (maybe even days, weeks, months) of hat-wearing and an inevitable level of self-assurance. Multiplying this by the right mind-set is the final step. Everyone has moments when they worry about what other people think of them, but if you can keep such thoughts at bay you'll find wearing a large hat supremely easy. To be honest, if you can banish them entirely you'll probably be ruling the world in a few years, renowned as a benevolent ruler who wore great hats.

Shortly after this it will start feeling more natural for you to wear hats every day, until you get to the point where your hand automatically reaches for a hat on your way out of the door and you feel naked without one. At this point there's no going back – you *are* a hat-wearer.

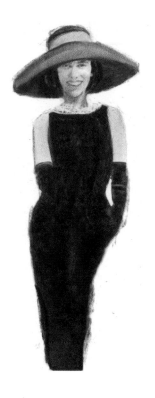

'The most important thing is to
enjoy your life, to be happy –
it's all that matters.'

Audrey Hepburn

GET THE LOOK:
The 1960s

When most people think hats, they think Audrey Hepburn – and more specifically, the iconic hat she wore in the 1961 film *Breakfast at Tiffany's*. It was the first film in which Audrey departed from her innocent, doe-eyed look of the Fifties, thereby triggering the fashion explosion of the Sixties.

The hat A wide-brimmed black hat is a good start and instantly lends you an Audrey aura, but the key point to this hat is the sweeping bow. These are more difficult to find in modern shops, so try looking for a thick cream bow you could tie around your hat instead – these can be found in normal fabric shops or craft shops.

The outfit A simple, sleek black dress is all you need. A mid-length one will suit those with longer legs.

The accessories Audrey completed this look with a pair of large sunglasses, and if you want to keep things simple that's all you'll need. If you'd prefer to pay close attention to detail, wear this with pearl earrings, black eyeliner and – if you're feeling confident – a pair of black gloves.

How to Avoid Hat-hair

—

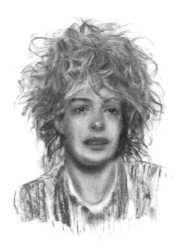

A problem often lamented is that of 'hat-hair', and it's one that's unfortunately largely unavoidable. Most of a threat to those with thin hair, symptoms include an advanced state of greasy hair, hair sticking to the head in an unflattering hat-shaped manner and – perhaps worst of all – the dreaded 'hat-fringe'. Little can be done to eliminate hat-fringe, as most hats press down on your hair, flattening it to the forehead and making it clump together most frustratingly.

There are obvious solutions to hat-hair, such as carrying dry shampoo or a hairbrush at all times, but these options might be impractical and require a good degree of organisation.

While these problems can't be solved outright, there are some hats that minimise the chances of developing hat-hair:

- THE BOATER A loose-fitting hat, thereby eliminating most hair-flattening incidents. It's also particularly good for fringes, as it tends to be worn tilted up, away from the forehead.

- THE BOWLER Although the traditional style of bowler hat is fairly fitted, its modern reincarnation sits in a similar way to the boater and is therefore a good alternative in colder weather.

- FLAT CAPS AND BERETS Both are small enough to do only minimal damage.

- PILLBOX HATS Excellent for smarter occasions.

- AVOID CLOCHE HATS Their closely fitted nature means they smooth your hair against your skull, and despite their many fine qualities this could be considered a major drawback.

The Ponytail Problem

—

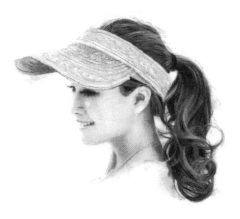

One of the most grievous issues faced by modern hat-wearers rears its head every summer: the Ponytail Problem.

It's hot. Your hair has created a thick, oppressive curtain of heat around your neck and all you want to do is throw it up into a ponytail. This, however, is quite impractical, as that lovely straw hat you were planning to wear won't fit comfortably with a ponytail in the way. Apart from cutting your hair off to avoid the problem forever (admittedly a tad drastic), options are limited.

THE BOATER

Once again the safest bet. Compact yet classic, it perches primly on top of your head, just about allowing room to sneak in a low ponytail if your hair is long enough.

VISORS

Not happy with a boater? The notion of a visor might seem absurd and offensive, but the perks of wearing one should not be ignored. While often considered painfully 1980s, it's possible to find elegant examples, and straw visors are simply perfect. One of these with a wide brim not only shades your face and shoulders from the sun and leaves room for the ponytail, but also evokes a sense of glamour and mystery that can't fail to turn heads.

SHORT OR FINE HAIR

This is easy to work with: tying a sleek bun at the nape of your neck is not only sophisticated, it also opens up further hat-wearing possibilities, with wide-brimmed straw hats once more becoming a viable choice.

What to Wear in the Wind

—

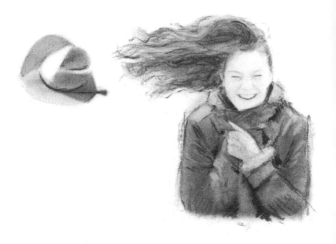

Wind is the hat's one great enemy. Any slight hint of a breeze can grab onto its brim and whisk it away – across roads, rivers, even onto train tracks. It's of course of the utmost importance to save said hat, but do of course bear in mind any consequent risk to your life. While the precise number of hat-related injuries remains unknown, it's sure to be fairly large, so here's a list of hats that will minimise any wind-based calamity:

- THE CLOCHE One of the most tightly fitting hats, the wind will have a hard time prising this from your clutches.

- THE BOWLER Traditional styles of bowler fit snugly and offer little risk, but even more modern styles have so small a brim that they're unlikely to be blown away.

- THE BERET A hat that can be worn in many ways, so simply style it to avoid attack.

- THE BEANIE An obvious choice. It's near impossible for it to be blown off.

Avoid at all costs:

- WIDE-BRIMMED HATS It almost goes without saying: if a breeze catches a wide-brimmed hat you'll have to run after the beautiful creation as if it were your own child.

- HATINATORS Precarious at the best of times, the hatinator is not one for blustery days. Of course, you might not have much choice, as they're so rarely worn, but if you're one to wear them often, maybe avoid the wind if you care anything for their well-being.

Spring

vs

Autumn

—

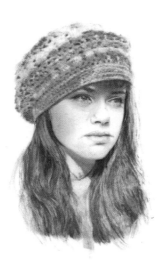

Flanking both the raw cold of winter and the blistering heat of summer (well, perhaps the vaguely tepid heat, at least) lie two tricky seasons for hat-wearers. It's overcast and warm enough to forgo a coat but still sufficiently cool that you need a jumper – do you venture out in a lively straw boater or keep to the Cossack? You might be rushed in the mornings and don't always have an extra half-hour to deliberate on the perfect hat, but fear not, here are a few suggestions:

SPRING

- Make the most of pale colours. You might be wearing a felt riding hat that could be too thick for the weather, but if it's in mint green it can't possibly look out of place.

- Pillbox hats are often also made of felt, but they cover so little of your head that they won't impede you with their bulk. As they usually come in bright colours, they can therefore make a good transition hat from winter into summer.

AUTUMN

- Berets are perfect to ease you back into a straw-hat-less existence after the summer, as they're small and light enough not to weigh you down as a heavy trapper hat might, but still thick enough to keep your head snug when needed.

- Flat caps are another compact and hassle-free option, but their thicker and more structured wool makes them more durable through the rainier seasons.

Hatcessories

—

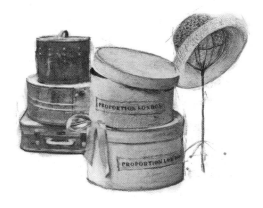

By this point you might have acquired an obscene number of hats, and for that you must be congratulated. But do you know how to properly take care of them? Which hatcessories to use and how? Consider the following tips...

STORAGE

The most pressing issue you'll face when your hat collection spills out of your wardrobe is where to start storing it. The best choice is a good old-fashioned hat stand to prevent your hats getting crumpled, but it's not always practical.

Hat boxes are the best alternative, and you can either get compact cardboard ones to fit under your bed or beautiful decorated ones that can be stacked up in the corner of your room. If that's not an option, it's admittedly trickier, but have you considered moving to a bigger house to accommodate your hats? No? Then how about hiding them in nooks and crannies around your house and screeching like a deranged animal if anyone tries to move them?

CLEANING

There will be times when your hats get dirty, but there's one simple solution to grubby felt. Find a hairbrush with soft bristles (a clothes brush would be perfect, but does anyone still own one?) and, holding your hat over steam from a pan of water or a kettle, brush at the dirt until it fades right away. Steam is also great for reshaping bent straw hats. And for getting a very sweaty face.

CARING FOR THE ELDERLY

When dealing with vintage hats you do need to exercise a certain degree of care. Feathers are likely to be extremely delicate, and old material can fray or get bent very easily. The best tip for a vintage hat is to put it in the freezer before wearing it for the first time. Most vintage shops are highly trustworthy, but you never know where that hat's been. If there do happen to be any creatures living inside it, a quick spell in the freezer should sort the problem out for good.

HATPINS

Hatpins are rarely used these days, but if you find yourself sick of walking around with your hand on your hat to stop it blowing away, maybe this is some-thing worth considering. Hatpins only work when your hair is up, of course, so it's not viable with every hat. Perhaps try it with a pillbox hat and your hair piled high underneath it. Look out for these in vintage shops and antiques markets.

Hatiquette

—

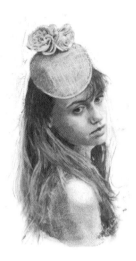

One further thing must be addressed before you fly off on your own, a competent hat-wearer: hatiquette.

WEARING HATS INDOORS

Whether it's polite or not to wear a hat indoors is an age-old question, for which there is no single answer, so a modern-day approach is best. It's not rude any more, and people are hardly likely to take offence, but let's be honest – you'd look a bit of an idiot.

Hats are more than a practical item of clothing, they're a fashion statement – indeed, they're a visual representation of the 'self' – but there's no logical sense in wearing them indoors. Chances of hat-hair incidents increase tenfold and it's simply not worth it.

HATS ON PUBLIC TRANSPORT

Wearing hats on trains, tubes or buses might be life-enhancing for you, but hatiquette dictates that if you're travelling in packed vehicles at peak times you really ought to make sure your hat isn't in the way. This might mean taking it off or even holding it high above the heads of others, but it's important not to provoke the wrath of your fellow travellers by wearing an aggressively inconvenient hat.

APPEALING TO THE MASSES

There should be no rules with hat-wearing, and you should not feel compelled to take any of this hatvice if you feel it goes against what your heart tells you. However, if you're wearing a top hat at a gig or a sombrero at the cinema, do yourself a favour and take it off. Hat-wearers might face others' confusion and mild irritation at their life choice, but if we can prevent outbreaks of violence, everyone would be a lot happier.

To tell the truth, hat-wearers rarely receive negative responses. Hats can become a talking point or conversation starter, and often elicit compliments from strangers in the street. People like seeing hats, talking about hats and maybe even thinking about them. The choice to become a hat-wearer is now on your own head, but that decision could very well have the power to change your life.

Popular
Hat Terms

—

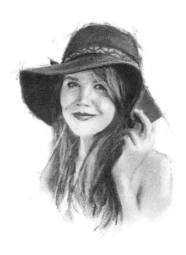

- HATASTROPHE Any hat-related disaster (e.g. the wind from a passing train blowing the hat off your head and onto the train tracks, rendering it unrescuable. Well, almost . . .).

- HATCESSORIES The tools needed for hat upkeep.

- HAT-LUST The sensation of purest envy felt when seeing another person's hat, combined with the desperate desire to make it your own.

- HATONEMENT A period of regret for a wrong done against a hat (e.g. sitting down and crushing it).

- HATROCITY A crime committed against a hat.

- HATSPIRATION The inspiration for a new hat that you simply *must* lay your hands on as soon as possible.

- HATTACK! When a (possibly inebriated) stranger steals a hat straight off your head.

- HATIQUETTE The etiquette of hat-wearing.

- HATTITUDE When you put on a hat and feel invincible.

- HATTRACTION Being attracted to someone ... but only because of their hat.

- HATTRIBUTES The benefits of wearing a hat.

- HATVISER Someone or something that gives advice on hats (e.g. '*The Art of Wearing Hats* is the greatest hatviser I've ever had!').

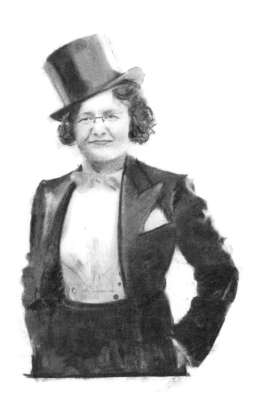

Final
Notes

N⚬5

'I have a hat. It is graceful and feminine and gives me a certain dignity, as if I were attending a state funeral or something. Someday I may get up enough courage to wear it, instead of carrying it.'

—

Erma Bombeck

Glossary

—

It's impossible to cover every single style of hat in this illustrious tome. Here are a few you might come across elsewhere, as well as a number of hat-related terms.

Aviator hat – Tight leather cap with earflaps, lined with sheepskin and worn with goggles by pilots in the pioneering years of aviation.

Baseball cap – Small cap made of cotton, with a stiff peak.

Bearskin – Very tall fur hat, usually worn in military ceremonies. Still worn occasionally in Britain today.

Beaver hat – Top hat made of felted beaver fur rather than silk and mainly worn by men in the 19th century.

Bicorne – Naval hat with the brim turned up at the front and back, creating two points at each side.

Bonnet – Soft cap made of silk or cotton, with a brim framing the face and tied beneath the chin with ribbons.

Breton – Naval-style cap often worn by fisherman and seafarers generally. It has a soft felt crown and short peak.

Brim – Edge of a hat, which runs all around it.

Cap – Hat with a peak at the front, rather than a brim.

Crown – Top of a hat.

Crush hat – Collapsible opera hat, developed so they could be put under chairs at the opera without getting damaged or blocking others' view.

Derby – Another name for a bowler hat.

Doff – Sign of respect when men raise their hat to a woman – 'To doff one's cap.'

Felt – Compressed wool used to make most hats.

Fez – Small hat of Ottoman origin with a flat top and without a brim.

Gibus – Collapsible top hat. Similar to the crush hat, this top hat could be collapsed and tucked under an arm when it got in the way.

Hat box – Large box to store hats in.

Hatpin – Long pin with an ornament at one end used to keep women's hats on their heads. Fastened by poking it through both hat and hair, which must be worn up for this to work.

Hat stand – Wooden or metal pole with spokes used to display or store hats.

Headscarf – Stretch of silk or cotton wrapped around the head and tied under the chin.

Hennin – Tall, pointed hat, sometimes with a veil, worn by women of rank in the 15th century.

Milliner – Someone who makes hats professionally.

Millinery – The art of making hats.

Panama hat – Hat made of Panama straw, woven in a similar style to the fedora.

St Catherine of Alexandria – French patron saint of milliners.

St Clement – English patron saint of milliners. Also said to have discovered felt.

Sombrero – Mexican straw or felt hat with a wide, upturned brim.

Stetson – Similar to a fedora, but sturdier and with a wider brim turned up at the sides. Made of felt or leather.

Tricorne – Naval hat turned in at the brim to create three points.

Visor – Peaked cap with no crown.

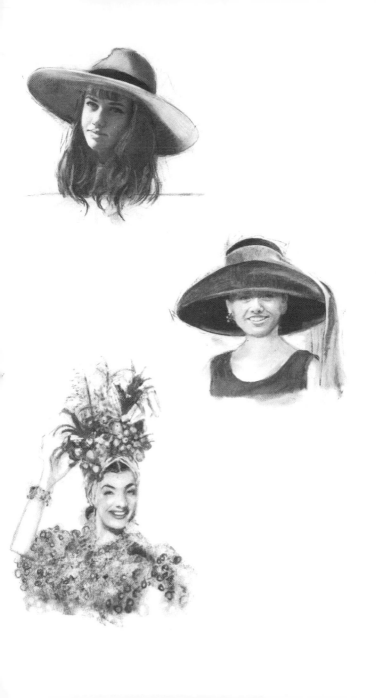

My Hat
Wish List

—

....
....
....
....
....
....
....
....
....
....
....
....
....
....
....
....
....

Recommended Hat Shops

—

Have you ever yearned for a specific hat, but not known where to find it? Listed here are some recommended hat shops. Of course, this only shows a handful – the perfect hat shop might be just around the corner, waiting for you to discover it ...

HIGH STREET

ACCESSORIZE Cloches, trilbies and fascinators.

DEBENHAMS Hatinators, fascinators and pillboxes.

H&M Berets, beanies and Cossacks.

JOHN LEWIS Hatinators, fascinators and pillboxes.

TOPSHOP/TOPMAN Fedoras, visors and wide-brims.

URBAN OUTFITTERS Panamas, beanies and snapbacks.

ONLINE

ASOS Using either the normal store or ASOS Marketplace, you'll be able to find so many hats here it's impossible to contemplate them all.

EBAY Try eBay for vintage-style hats and rare hats at very good prices.

ETSY If you're looking for something really unique, Etsy can provide you with a multitude of handmade hats and headdresses for every occasion.

HATS AND CAPS This website has an almost inexhaustible array of hats and caps for men, women and children, sorted by style or brand to make it easier. You might find it hard to leave ...

VINTAGE SHOPS

BEYOND RETRO (ONLINE AND ON THE HIGH STREET) With branches in England and Sweden, and an excellent online store, Beyond Retro is one of the biggest vintage suppliers, trusted for both quality and quirkiness.

CAMDEN MARKET Famed for its huge variety of stalls and shops (and admittedly a big tourist attraction), browsing through Camden Market will undoubtedly unearth some unique treasures.

CHESHIRE STREET, SHOREDITCH, LONDON Almost every other shop on this street is vintage. If you want to blitz your budget in one go, this is the place for you. There are enough hats here to fulfil your wildest fantasies, and if you still don't find one you're right on the doorstep of Brick Lane and Spitalfields Market – prepare yourself for some serious perusing.

JUDY'S AFFORDABLE VINTAGE FAIR This vintage fair is perfect for beginners and seasoned vintage shoppers alike. Constantly touring around Britain, it offers a mind-boggling number of dresses, shirts, brooches, posters, trinkets, bags and, of course, hats. Most importantly, it's not lying about being affordable.

ROKIT (ONLINE AND ON THE HIGH STREET) Rokit has four branches in London and a huge online store. Their selection of hats and headdresses is simply fantastic.

THE POP BOUTIQUE (COVENT GARDEN, LON— DON) This shop may be small, but it is affordable and always hides a gem or two within. It does have a small website, but is definitely worth a visit if possible.

INDEPENDENT HAT SHOPS

CHRISTYS' LONDON If you're looking for something supremely refined, try Christys'. Their website has a section on hatiquette, so you know you can trust them.

LAIRD & CO. Based in London and Cambridge, Laird & Co. supply exquisite hats to the well-dressed gentleman (while of course catering to women as well).

LOCK & CO. With a long history of supplying hats, Lock & Co. have an impressive selection available, along with hatcessories to go with them.

THE MADHATTER BOOKSHOP Hats and books. What more do you need? This brilliant shop is based in Oxfordshire but also has a website for those who can't get to it.

Index
by
Season

—

Acknowledgements

—

First, I'd like to thank the pink fluffy beret – given to me on my thirteenth birthday – that inspired my ludicrous hat obsession. Thanks too to my family, for enduring the past twenty-plus years of my existence, and without whose regular ridicule I would not be the semi-sane person I am today; in particular, my esteemed aunt/illustrator, Sian Tezel, for her tireless enthusiasm and unflinching flattery regarding this book.

Thank you to Emily Barrett, who edited the manuscript with the style and boundless insight of a true hat admirer, and to Lucy Sykes-Thompson, whose cover design is so gorgeous my mother didn't complain about the pink. Finally, thank you to the entire HarperCollins sales team, whom I have threatened repeatedly in the hope that they'll be scared into selling the book – especially to Laura Fletcher, Jay Cochrane, Sarah Collett, Laura Garrod, Tom Dunstan and Dominic Rigby, because without you this would probably never have stood a chance. Thank you in advance for making *The Art of Wearing Hats* a worldwide bestseller.

About the Author

—

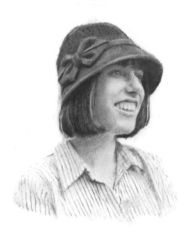

Helena Sheffield is the proud owner of somewhere over forty hats. While she currently works in publishing, she expects to venture into professional hat-wearing very shortly, with her first aim being to move into an office big enough for all her hats. Rumours about her next book, *Who Wants to Be a Milliner: How to Make Money from Hat-Wearing*, remain unconfirmed.